The IMMUNE FACTOR

DISCOVER THE MIRACLE OF YOUR IMMUNE SYSTEM— LIVE DISEASE FREE

BY

DR. MICHAEL T. MURRAY

North America's Leading Naturopathic Physician

D0036702

MIND PUBLISHING INC.

Copyright © 2001

Illustrations: Ernie Thomsen
Photography: Stephen Rank/Ed Park
Design: Stephen Rank

For information contact:
Natural MediFAQs
www.naturalmedifaqs.com
info@naturalmedifaqs.com

ISBN

First printing August 2001

Printed in Canada

*NOTE: ECHINAMIDE™ is a trademark of Natural Factors Nutritional Products Ltd. and is used when referring to that specific echinacea product. For readability the ™ will not be used throughout the body text of this book.

Overview

This book highlights the development of a significant advancement in one of the most popular herbal medicines in the world – echinacea. In the last few years, there has been a tremendous renaissance in the use and appreciation of herbal medicine. In addition to echinacea, other herbs like St. John's wort and Ginkgo biloba have become household words in North America. Surprisingly, improvements in technology have ultimately been responsible for this increase in the popularity of traditional medicines. Advancements in science have made it possible to know better how to grow a plant, when to harvest it, how to concentrate an extract for maximum concentration of medicinal components, and how those medicinal components work in the human body to promote health. *The Immune Factor* details the evolution of echinacea from a folk remedy to a well-accepted, natural approach to boosting immune function.

This book is dedicated to the
life-long work of Roland Gahler, who is
fulfilling his dream of setting standards for
herbal research and effectiveness.

CONTENTS

About the Author

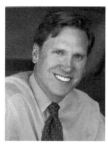 Michael T. Murray, ND, is widely regarded as one of the world's leading authorities on natural medicine. He is a graduate, faculty member and member of the Board of Trustees of Bastyr University in Seattle, Washington. He is co-author of *A Textbook of Natural Medicine*, the definitive textbook on naturopathic medicine for physicians, as well as the consumer version, *The Encyclopedia of Natural Medicine*. He has written more than 20 other books including his latest, *Dr. Murray's Total Body Tune-Up*. Total cumulative sales of his books exceed 2 million copies.

For twenty years, Dr. Murray has compiled a massive database of scientific studies from medical literature—more than 50,000 articles on the effectiveness of diet, vitamins, minerals, glandular extracts, herbs, and other natural measures in maintaining health and treating disease. He has been instrumental in bringing many effective natural products to North America, including Glucosamine Sulfate, St. John's Wort extract, Ginkgo biloba extract and others. Dr. Murray has dedicated his life to educating physicians, patients and the general public on the tremendous healing power of nature. He is a popular lecturer for the public and professionals, and he has appeared on hundreds of radio and TV programs.

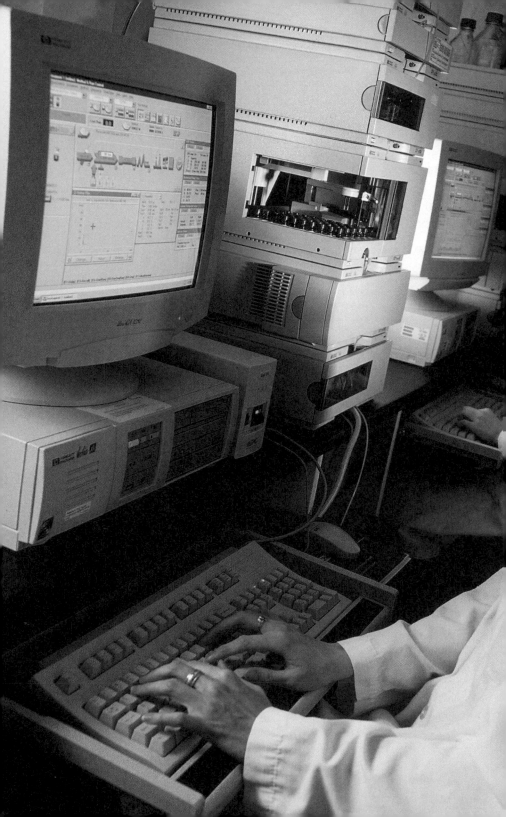

Science Fuels an Herbal Renaissance

Since the early 1980s there has been a tremendous increase in the use and appreciation of herbal medicine in North America. I have termed this process the Herbal Renaissance. Most people are surprised to learn that the primary fuel for this increased popularity of herbal medicine is scientific research. During the last 20 to 30 years there has been a virtual explosion of scientific information concerning the medicinal use of plants. Through science we now have a better understanding of how a particular herb might work to promote health. We also now know how to grow a plant for highest medicinal effect, when to harvest it and how to concentrate the medicinal components in extracts.

Some people interested in herbal medicine are turned off by the word "science", but by definition "science" refers to "possession of knowledge, as distinguished from ignorance or misunderstanding." Scientific knowledge is based upon the scientific method, meaning that the understanding is based on data collected through observation and experiment. It must be kept in mind, that while science is evolutionary, the underlying natural laws it seeks to explain or clarify are constant. In other words, gravity existed long before Sir Isaac Newton was around to explain it. In regards to herbs, their medicinal properties existed prior to our discovery or understanding.

I am stressing the importance of science here because it underscores the development of Echinamide and serves as the basis for this discussion of herbs and science. Echinamide is the trademarked name of a unique patented, super-extracted echinacea product developed and marketed by Natural Factors Nutritional Products.

The personal and financial commitment of Roland Gahler, President of Natural Factors, and the persistence and expertise of his science team, have led to the development of what is now considered by many leading authorities on echinacea to be the ultimate echinacea product on the market anyplace in the world—Echinamide. Grown under certified organic standards at Factor Farms, Echinamide is produced under careful control by Natural Factors; from planting the organic seedlings, through harvesting and extraction, to distribution on to the shelves of your local health food store.

The Immune Factor highlights the uniqueness of this echinacea plant and product and explains exactly how Natural Factors' science and medical advisory teams have used scientific methods to actually improve echinacea. Here is a summary of these important developments:

Improved Analytical Techniques

- The team developed appropriate chemical analysis techniques to isolate and measure the specific substances (phytochemicals) within Echinacea purpurea responsible for its immune enhancing effects.

Better Growing Conditions

- Natural Factors has determined the optimum growing conditions for Echinacea purpurea, using 100% organic methods, to consistently yield the highest levels of active compounds.

More Precise Harvesting

- By determining the level of active compounds throughout the growing cycle, Natural Factors is able to harvest the echinacea at the most ideal time–when it is highest in active compounds.

Use of Only Fresh Herb Material

- Natural Factors uses fresh echinacea. Up to 30 percent of the active compounds can be lost in the drying processes used by many other growers and manufacturers.

Advanced Extraction Techniques

• Many key compounds in echinacea are typically lost during the extraction phase or are left behind due to inappropriate extraction methods. Natural Factors has developed a patented extraction technique to produce Echinamide, with the highest levels and broadest range of active compounds available.

Improved Experimental Models

• Natural Factors worked with leaders in pharmacology to develop the experimental models designed to better understand and measure the immune enhancing effects of echinacea.
(See research results later in this book).

Proper Clinical Evaluation

• The encouraging results from preliminary studies with Echinamide are being followed by detailed clinical studies at major universities.

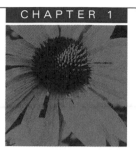

CHAPTER 1

A Vision of the Future

I truly believe that the medicine of the future will include, to a very large extent, the medicine of the past—particularly time-tested herbal medicines like echinacea. There is a trend towards using substances found in nature such as foods, food components, herbs and herbal compounds. There is also an increase in the understanding and use of naturally occurring compounds found in the human body, such as interferon, interleukin, insulin and human growth hormone. More and more researchers are discovering the tremendous healing properties of these natural compounds and their advantages over synthetic medicines, drugs and surgery in the treatment of many health conditions.

The use of echinacea for infectious conditions is undoubtedly becoming as popular here in North America as it is in Europe. My hope is that echinacea will become even more popular, and will play a significant role in reducing our population's excessive reliance on, and abuse of, antibiotics. Over-dependence on antibiotics is creating many long term problems, such as the development of "superbugs" resistant to currently available antibiotics. According to many experts, including those at the World Health Organization, we are coming dangerously close to arriving at a "post-antibiotic era" where many infectious diseases will become resistant to all conventional antibiotics.

My view of this challenge is that it will force conventional medical practitioners and scientists to take a closer look at natural ways to enhance the body's resistance against infection. If they do so, I believe they will discover the healing power of nature and the magic of such plants as echinacea in boosting immune function. There is a growing body of knowledge that supports the use of whole foods and nutritional supplements in the maintenance of health and treatment of disease. In terms of enhancing resistance to infection, a great deal can be done using diet, nutritional supplements, herbal products, and other natural therapies.

The Infection Equation

The infection equation is like a mathematical equation where one plus two equals three. In the infection equation the interaction of the host's immune system with the infecting organism determines the equation's outcome. Each day each of us is exposed to organisms that have the potential to make us sick, yet we don't always fall prey to these "bugs" because our immune system is generally stronger than the organism. If the

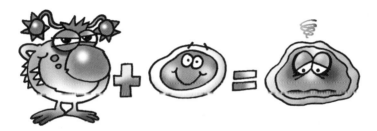

"bug" is extremely powerful, or our immune system is compromised, an infection can occur.

For too long modern medicine has ignored the role of immune function in the infection equation. Conventional medicine has been obsessed with the nature of the "beast", the infecting agent, rather than the condition of the host and its defense factors.

This obsession began with Louis Pasteur, the 19th century physician and researcher who played a major role in the development of the germ theory. Pasteur theorized that infectious organisms cause most diseases and much of Pasteur's life was dedicated to finding substances that would kill infecting organisms. Pasteur and others who pioneered effective treatments of infectious diseases have given us a great deal, for which we should be grateful, however, there is more to this equation than the nature of the "beast".

Another 19th century French scientist, Claude Bernard, also made major contributions to medical understanding. Only Bernard had a different view of health and disease. Bernard believed that the state of a person's internal environment was more important in preventing or responding to disease than the invading organism (commonly called a pathogen). Bernard believed that the susceptibility of the host to infection was more important than the nature of the germ. Logically, he believed that physicians should focus more of their attention on making this internal terrain a very inhospitable place for disease.

Bernard's theory led to some rather interesting studies, including some that would seem pretty crazy to any advocate of the germ theory. One of the most interesting studies was conducted by a Russian scientist named Elie Metchnikoff, the discovery of white blood cells. He and his research associates consumed cultures containing millions of cholera bacteria. Yet none of them developed cholera. The reason? Their immune systems were not compromised. Metchnikoff believed, like Bernard, that the correct way to deal with infectious disease was to focus on enhancing the body's defenses.

During the last part of their lives, Pasteur and Bernard engaged in scientific discussions comparing the virtues of the germ theory and Bernard's perspective on the internal terrain. On his deathbed, Pasteur said: "Bernard was right. The pathogen is nothing. The terrain is everything."

Unfortunately, Pasteur's legacy, the obsession with the pathogen, has become predominant in modern medicine and the importance of the "terrain" has been forgotten by many. But the perspective is slowly changing. This book looks at the role echinacea can play in enhancing immune function to make your body's terrain extremely inhospitable to infecting organisms.

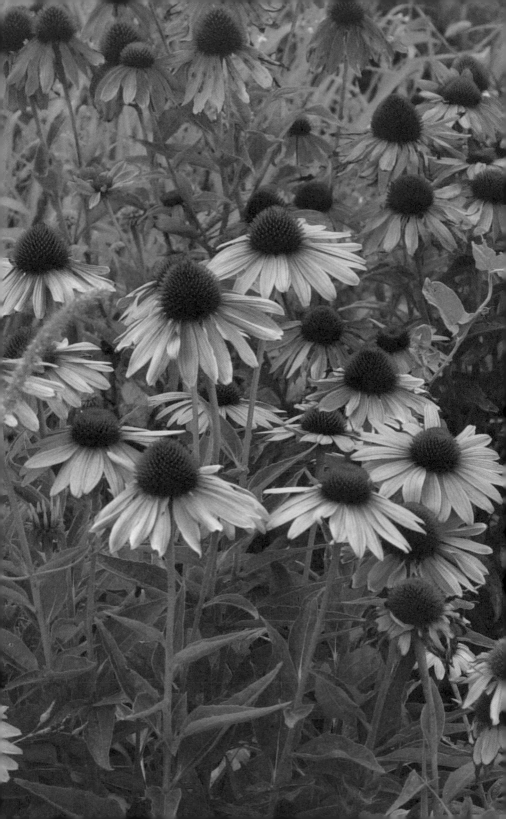

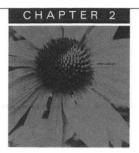

CHAPTER 2

The Evolution of Echinacea

I n every native culture around the globe medicinal plants have been used and valued, and often one in particular has been held in the highest reverence. Many of these plants are now household names: herbs such as ginseng, kava, saw palmetto and, of course echinacea.

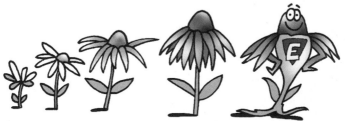

In North America the medicinal plant that has garnered the greatest respect among Native Americans is echinacea, the purple coneflower. This perennial plant is native to the North American Midwest, from Saskatchewan to Texas, and has been traditionally used by Native Americans against more illnesses than any other plant. Externally it was used for the healing of wounds, burns, abscesses, and insect bites while internally it was used for infections, toothache and joint pain; and as an antidote for rattlesnake bite!

When did "Western Medicine" Discover Echinacea?

Echinacea became quite familiar to settlers during the 18th and 19th centuries. Its popularity soared when a commercial product containing echinacea was introduced to Americans in 1870 by H.C.F. Meyer, a German lay healer, who recommended it as a wonder cure called "Meyer's blood purifier." Just like the natives, Meyer recommended it for almost every conceivable malady. There were in fact numerous case reports of echinacea successfully treating snake bite, typhus, diphtheria and other infections. One of the most interesting aspects of the history of echinacea is that modern research helps us understand and validate this herb's historical use as a "blood purifier." Although this term is now antiquated, based on recent scientific studies there is ample evidence that echinacea does, in fact, help purify the blood. It stimulates the cells responsible for clearing foreign material from the blood, while it rids the body of viruses, bacteria, cancer cells and other particulate matter.

Although many physicians in the late 1800s and early 1900s began to investigate and use echinacea as a serious medicine, in 1909 the Council on Pharmacy and Chemistry of the American Medical Association refused to recognize echinacea as an active drug. They stated: "In view of the lack of any scientific scrutiny of the claims made for it, echinacea is deemed unworthy of further consideration until more reliable evidence is presented in its favor." Despite this opposition, echinacea was included in the National Formulary of the United States and remained there until 1950.

Abandoned then Rediscovered

With the development of antibiotics and other modern medicines, the popularity of echinacea in the US waned (except amongst naturopathic physicians) until around 1980. Then echinacea was "rediscovered" due to increased consumer interest in immune system disorders such as chronic candidiasis, chronic fatigue syndrome, AIDS and cancer.

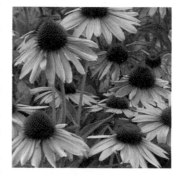

Although interest in echinacea decreased in America between the 1930s and 1980s, European physicians set out to provide the kind of evidence the American Medical Association had called for back in 1909. One of the first European studies was a 1932 study by Gerhard Madaus that demonstrated immune-enhancing effects of a preparation from the fresh juice of the aerial portion of E. purpurea. This study was followed by development of commercial echinacea products and a great deal of scientific study.

In fact, the chemistry, pharmacology and clinical applications of echinacea have now been the subject of well over 300 scientific studies.

Many Different Echinacea Species

Eleven species of echinacea have been identified. They are named with an E for echinacea and then the Latin species identifier. For example *E. angustifolia*, *E. purpurea*, and *E. pallida* which are the most popular species used in herbal medicine.

Echinacea derives its name from the Greek echinos, meaning sea urchin, referring to the prickly scales of the flower's dried seed head. All echinacea species have this characteristic scaly cone-shaped head, but they tend to differ in the color or shape of the flowers, the color of the pollen or the overall height of the plant. For example, *E. purpurea* has wider purple flowers and grows much higher (up to 5.5 feet) than *E. angustifolia*. There is no clear clinical evidence that any particular species offers advantages over the others although *E. purpurea* is emerging as the preferred species due to its higher levels of key active ingredients. Specifically, Natural Factors has chosen to use the fresh, above-ground portion of *E. purpurea* as the source material for Echinamide based not only on its chemical profile, but also preliminary evidence of superior effects on various functions of white blood cells.

What is Echinamide?

In case you missed it in the introduction, Echinamide is the trademarked name of a unique patented, super-extracted echinacea product developed and marketed by Natural Factors. The herb is grown under certified organic standards at Factor Farms and Echinamide production is controlled by Natural Factors through all its aspects—from planting the organic seedlings, through harvesting and extraction, to its appearance on the shelves of your local health food store. The result is that Natural Factors has developed an echinacea product with the highest levels and broadest range of active compounds available.

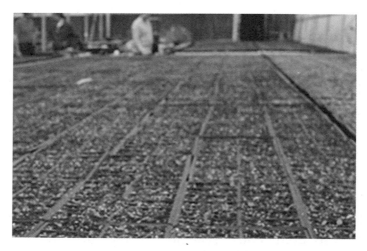

Echinamide starts with organic seedlings of E. purpurea grown
under controlled circumstances by Natural Factors.

Phytochemicals that Boost Immunity: Why does Echinamide work?

Echinacea's most important phytochemicals, a name for active plant constituents, fall into six categories:

1 *polysaccharides*

2 *cichoric acid and other caffeic acid derivatives*

3 *alkylamides*

4 *flavonoids*

5 *essential oils and*

6 *glycoproteins.*

These compounds, and how they affect immune system function, are discussed in the next chapter. Not all echinacea − either in the field or in a bottle − contains all these components and some powdered products don't contain ANY active ingredients! One of the unique features of Echinamide echinacea is that it contains ALL these components and is especially high in *E. purpurea's* three key actives: polysaccharides, cichoric acid and alkylamides. In fact, Echinamide has guaranteed high levels of these three compounds, unlike any other echinacea product on the market. This is because of its unique, patented multiple extraction process and the research that has gone into producing Echinamide.

Since echinacea contains a wide assortment of chemical constituents with immune enhancing effects, it is important for manufacturers to insure sufficient levels of these active compounds. Unfortunately, most echinacea products on the market do not specify the levels of active compounds because they have not been analyzed for them. When manufacturers do state the level of a particular marker compound, most consumers fail to realize that concentrating only one particular active compound of echinacea can result in a loss of other constituents, and all of the herb's synergistic effects. For example, some manufacturers standardize for "total phenolic content" or the compound echinacoside. However, recent studies have found these preparations may have some antioxidant properties, but have no effect on enhancing immune function in experimental animal studies.[1]

What is a "Synergistic Effect"?

One of the most interesting phenomena in nature is synergy. In the case of echinacea, it appears that individual immune enhancing compounds produce

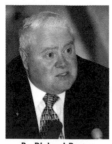

Dr. Richard Barton
University of British Columbia

significant effects, but when they are combined in meaningful amounts there is an added or multiplied effect much greater than the individual components have separately. The immune enhancing components of echinacea work together in a harmonious fashion to produce the phenomena of immune building synergy. In other words, $1 + 1 + 1 = 6$.

Echinamide is unique in that it not only has standardized levels of active compounds, they are in ratios that have been shown to produce this synergistic effect. It is not enough to be high in any one particular component of echinacea, for maximum benefit it is very important that the product contain all of the active components in their natural and most effective ratios. And, that is exactly what makes Echinamide different from all other echinacea products.

Under the direction of Dr. Richard Barton of the University of British Columbia, Natural Factors has developed the necessary scientific methods to properly analyze echinacea as well as to ensure that each batch of Echinamide contains consistent, standardized levels of active components.

The German Research Connection

In the early part of the 1900s there was considerable research on echinacea in the United States. However the growth of the pharmaceutical industry, coupled with a long-standing bias against herbal medicine by

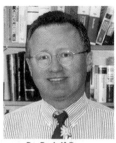

Dr. Rudolf Bauer
Heinrich-Heine University

American physicians, led to discontinuation of this research in North America. Large American pharmaceutical firms chose to focus their research on isolated and chemically modified compounds that could be patented. In contrast, European policies on herbal medicines made it economically feasible for companies to research and develop "phytopharmaceuticals" (plant-based drugs). Plus, in contrast to the United States, herbal medicine is an intrinsic part of the culture and history in Germany so physicians there were less biased against echinacea.

Beginning with Madaus' work in 1937, German researchers have led the way in our understanding of echinacea (as well as many other plants such as St. John's wort and Ginkgo biloba). While professor Hildebert Wagner of the University of Munich has also played a major role in echinacea research, the real leader in the scientific understanding of echinacea is Dr. Rudolf Bauer of the Heinrich-Heine University in Düsseldorf, Germany. Dr. Bauer has conducted and published more research on echinacea than any other person. His research has been critical not only to the understanding of echinacea but also to its growing acceptance as an immune enhancing agent. Much of the information on echinacea presented in the following chapter originated with Dr. Bauer. He is, without question, the world's leading

Dr. Bauer has conducted, reviewed and published dozens of scientific studies on E. purpurea and is considered a world authority on the subject.

authority on echinacea and was a key advisor in the research that has produced Echinamide.

Dr. Bauer on Echinamide

Dr. Rudolf Bauer is the world's foremost authority on echinacea. His involvement in Echinamide research has been extremely valuable. According to Dr. Bauer, "Echinamide is unique in that it has certain standardized levels of polysaccharides, cichoric acid and alkylamides."

Regarding the research conducted with Echinamide, Dr. Bauer says, "This new data, which has produced pharmacological results, cannot be transferred to other products. It is only Echinamide that was used and only Echinamide has been proven to create these results. Past research has been relatively useless because it failed to work with a standardized, consistent echinacea extract. But Echinamide is such an extract."

There are more than 300 echinacea products sold in the world, only one with the unique phytochemical profile of Echinamide.

Haven't Other Echinacea Products Been Tested?

Yes, but there is a serious problem when you look closely at echinacea research – the lack of quality control in defining the echinacea product used has led to inconsistent results. While some studies have been positive, others have not. The main reason may be that

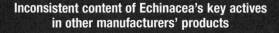

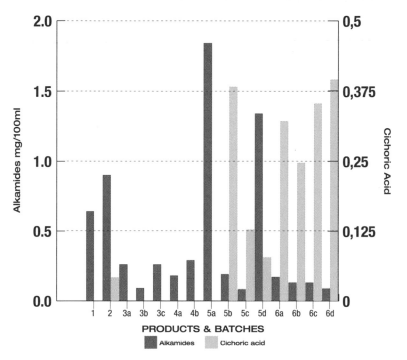

In research by Dr. R. Bauer, remarkable variances were found between the levels of cichoric acid and alkylamides in different preparations from the same manufacturers, and even from the same batches of E. purpurea expressed juices.

(a, b, c, etc. indicate different batches from the same manufacturer)

No such variances exist with ECHINAMIDE extract.

the echinacea extracts or products used in these studies contained unspecified levels of active ingredients.

Therefore, there was no way to be sure that the echinacea product used contained sufficient levels of these key compounds to produce any significant immune enhancing activity. Since the effectiveness of any herbal product (or drug for that matter) depends upon consistently delivering an effective dosage of active compounds, it is likely that an insufficient dosage of active compounds was used in many of the studies.

Chemical analysis of commercial echinacea preparations has demonstrated tremendous variation in the levels of key compounds even within the same product from batch to batch. For example, when Dr. Bauer analyzed various commercial echinacea products he found that there was tremendous variation in the level of cichoric acid with most products containing either none or very little.

Why are Echinacea Products so Different from One to Another?

Most manufacturers do not employ the necessary quality control tests required to ensure that their echinacea is properly planted, harvested at the exact time for maximal levels of all active compounds and processed for maximum protection of key active ingredients.

It is imperative that the echinacea be treated properly after harvesting. First of all, it is absolutely essential to use fresh plant material versus the dried plant or roots that most manufacturers use. Studies indicate that a significant amount of the active ingredients are destroyed in the drying process.[2-5] Processing time is also very important. If the fresh plant material is not processed immediately, the content of several key components—especially cichoric acid and alkylamides—will be low (as much as 80 percent of actives will be lost).

It is also essential that extraction occur under ideal conditions. Natural Factors is committed to finding the best conditions for extraction of echinacea destined to become Echinamide, so the plants will yield the highest possible levels of active components. The company determines the best portion of the plant to use, as well as the right temperature, length of time for extraction, and right concentrations for alcohol and water. Since the active components have different solubility characteristics (some are more soluble in water, others are more soluble in alcohol), different extractions are conducted to concentrate the active compounds. By blending these concentrated and tested extracts, Natural Factors produces Echinamide.

Primary Uses of Echinacea

Based upon currently existing clinical research, the clinical applications of echinacea include:

- Treatment of the common cold and other viral respiratory tract infections.

- Possible prevention of the common cold and viral respiratory tract infections.

- Treatment of temporary immune deficiency and increased susceptibility to infections, for example, children in daycare or nurseries, adults experiencing undue stress, or sport-induced immunodeficiency.

- Supportive therapy to enhance the effectiveness of antibiotics in bacterial infections.

- Chemotherapy and radiation-induced immune suppression.

- Herpes simplex infections.

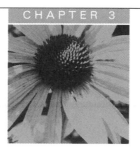

CHAPTER 3

ECHINAMIDE™ and the Immune System

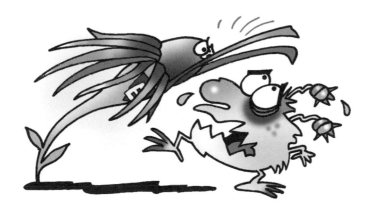

B efore we can truly appreciate the magic that echinacea exerts on enhancing and balancing immune function, we must understand some of the key "players" in the immune system. With such an understanding, you will discover that echinacea can exert a broad-spectrum of effects on the immune system thanks to its various active components affecting different aspects of immune function.

The immune system is the body's chief defense system. It is beautifully designed to protect the body against foreign attackers such as germs, viruses, bacteria, and other creatures generally known as pathogens. The human immune system is composed of the lymphatic vessels and organs (thymus, spleen, tonsils, and lymph nodes), white blood cells, specialized cells residing in various tissues, and specialized proteins in the blood.

White blood cells are the foot soldiers of the immune system. There are two main types of white blood cells: granulocytes and lymphocytes (-cyte means "cell").

Granulocytes are so called because they contain granules, or tiny sacs, that store chemicals. Granulocytes engulf and destroy bacteria, cancerous cells and dead particles by releasing enzymes from their granules that break the particle into smaller harmless parts.

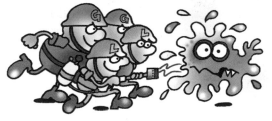

Granulocytes engulf and destroy bacteria

Lymphocytes are a type of white blood cell that does not "eat" the invaders. Instead their strategy is to disable them with special destructive chemicals. Lymphocytes play a central role in fighting viral infections and cancer.

Echinacea and the White Blood Cells

Echinacea exerts multiple effects on white blood cell function. Remember echinacea's historical use as a "blood purifier"? Well, nowadays, we know that the body's chief garbage collection and elimination system is part of the immune system called the reticuloendothelial system. (Whew! That's a mouthful.) Let's call it the RES. The RES comprises white blood cells in the spleen, lymph nodes, liver, bone marrow, lungs and intestines.

The RES is designed to purify the blood indirectly by filtering lymphatic fluid—a fluid that contains primarily waste products from cellular activity—as it passes through the lymph nodes. Lymph nodes are small, soft, bean-shaped nodules clustered in various parts of the body, such as the neck, armpit, and groin. Lymph nodes are connected via lymphatic vessels that run parallel to our blood vessels. Lymph fluid flows through a lymph node in one direction, so that the fluid leaving the node is always cleaner than the fluid that enters it.

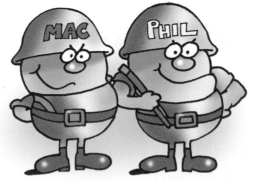

Macrophage and neutrophils are two types
of infection-fighting white blood cells

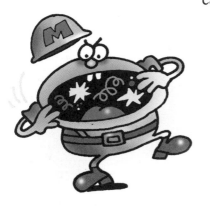

Macrophage means Big Eater

The lymph nodes and other components filter lymph by calling on special white blood cells called macrophages, Latin for "big eaters." These large and apparently hungry cells engulf and destroy particles such as old blood cells, bacteria, viruses and even cancer cells through a process known as phagocytosis. Another type of white blood cell capable of phagocytosis is called a neutrophil.

Macrophages are found throughout the body, especially in the liver, spleen and lymph nodes and macrophages that circulate in the blood are known as monocytes. The macrophage is so important to the RES, that this garbage collecting and eliminating system is also known as the monocyte-macrophage system.

"Swollen Glands?" The Lymph Node vs Infection Phenomenon

When foreign materials are recognized in the lymph fluid, the lymph nodes enlarge as they produce and supply additional white blood cells to help fight infection. During an infection, the nodes are working overtime to collect and destroy infectious agents. That's why they often swell when an infection starts to attack.

Echinacea to the Rescue!

One of the key ways echinacea enhances immune function is by stimulating the ability of macrophages to engulf and destroy particles.[1,6-8] By enhancing the activity of these "garbage collectors" of the body, the blood is essentially purified.

The specific components of echinacea responsible for this effect are the polysaccharides, alkylamides, and cichoric acid. While each component is effective alone, the greatest degree of immune stimulation is noted when the three active components are used in combination in the form of Echinamide.[9] This was proven in research conducted by Dr. Tapan Basu of the University of Alberta, Canada, using Echinamide because of its consistent, standardized nature. What Dr. Basu demonstrated was the phenomena of synergy along with a clear dose-dependent effect. In other words, Dr. Basu demonstrated that the immune enhancing effects were greater with all three actives working together than any individual active and that the higher the dose of Echinamide, the greater the effect on macrophage function.

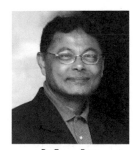

Dr. Tapan Basu
University of Alberta

Dr. Basu and others have also demonstrated that, besides enhancing the ability of the macrophages to engulf and destroy foreign molecules, the active components of echinacea also help the macrophages detect foreign matter in the blood and signal the other parts of the immune system to mount an attack.

This signal is in the form of chemical messengers. More than a dozen different factors have been identified that enable the body to communicate internally when an invasion occurs. Interestingly, some of these messengers have been developed as drugs through genetic engineering. Two such elements are interleukin-1 (IL-1) and granulocyte colony stimulating factor (GCSF). While these purified agents show promise as immune boosters, especially in cancer patients, they are extremely expensive at this time. Echinamide could be an effective and reasonably priced, safe alternative to these expensive drugs.

Echinacea and the Lymphocytes (not a rock band)

Echinacea also effects the lymphocytes, white blood cells that act as the immune system's "special forces", combination Green Berets and Navy Seals. Lymphocytes use special destructive chemicals, search-and-destroy tactics and highly sophisticated communication techniques. About eighty percent of your lymphocytes are "T cells" that mature in the thymus gland—the major "base camp" for the immune team—which consists of two pinkish lobes in the upper chest. T cells are responsible for an important immune response known as cell-mediated immunity. Some T cells ("killer T cells") destroy invaders by attaching to them and causing them to break apart.

Other T cells ("helper T cells") release special chemical messengers, calling other types of immune cells to the scene of attack and encouraging them to do their job. Once the mission is accomplished, another type of cell, the "suppressor T cell", arrives and issues orders to stop the attack.

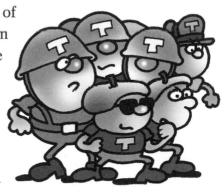

T-cells destroy invaders

Cell-mediated immunity is extremely important in providing resistance to infection by mold-like bacteria, yeast (including Candida albicans), fungi, parasites, and viruses (including herpes simplex, Epstein-Barr virus, and viruses that cause hepatitis). If a person is suffering from an infection by these organisms, it's a good indication that their cell-mediated immunity is not functioning up to par. Cell-mediated immunity is also critical in protecting against the development of cancer, autoimmune disorders such as rheumatoid arthritis, and allergies. Not surprisingly, echinacea has been used to treat all of these conditions.

The other major type of lymphocyte is the B cell. These cells are responsible for the immune response called humoral immunity. Like alert sentries, B cells recognize the specific types of foreign particles present, including bacteria, yeast and viruses. These foreign particles are referred to as antigens. In response to an antigen, B cells produce an antibody. Antibodies (also

41

known as immunoglobulins) are special protein molecules that attach to antigens. If the antigen is on the surface of an invading organism (a pathogen, or disease causing organism), the antibody will bind to it and lead to its destruction. Each antibody must be tailor-made to fit the specific invader, so it takes a few days for B lymphocytes to crank out enough of them to be effective. In contrast, the cell-mediated response by T cells is immediate.

Old Soldiers Keep Fighting

Helper T cells and B lymphocytes have relatively long lives and excellent memories. The next time an invader tries to attack the cells, they remember how they mounted the previous defense. T cells send messages to B cells, ordering them to produce the same type of antibodies that worked before. Basically, this memory process translates into lifelong immunity and is the same mechanism by which vaccines work.

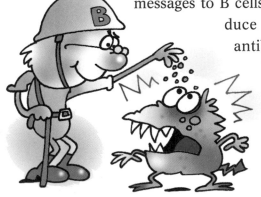

Some T-cells have long lives

Vaccines produce a simulated infection by introducing the antigen without a viable organism. The body mounts an attack just as if it was infected. However, unlike actual infections, many vaccines do not produce lifelong immunity and "booster shots" may be required for the vaccine to continue to be effective. Also, some organisms, like flu viruses, outsmart the body's defenses by mutating.

CELL-MEDIATED (T CELL) IMMUNITY Protects Against:	HUMORAL (B CELL) IMMUNITY Protects Against:
Most viruses (e.g., herpes simplex)	Some viruses (e.g., measles)
Most mycoplasma (e.g., tuberculosis)	Most bacteria (e.g., strep and staph)
Most yeast (e.g., candidiasis)	Most parasites (e.g., giardia)

The remaining types of lymphocytes are the natural killer cells. Natural killer (NK) cells got their name because they can destroy cells that have become cancerous or infected with viruses. They are especially important because they provide vital protection against the development and spread of cancer.

Echinamide on the Front Lines

Echinacea affects lymphocytes in an indirect and direct manner.[10-12] The indirect manner is via enhancing macrophage function. Macrophages assist lymphocytes in many ways. For example, it is the macrophage's job to grab hold of the organism and present it to a lymphocyte for "processing". In this respect the macrophage is a lot like the military police apprehending a suspect and the lymphocyte is like the judge at a court martial deciding how the suspect should be treated. By being better able to apprehend the culprit, there is a better chance that it will be brought to justice.

Echinacea directly affects lymphocytes by literally turning them on. This action is referred to as "nonspecific T-cell activation". By doing this, echinacea leads to a cascade of effects including improved overall function of the lymphocytes and secretion of many immune enhancing chemicals known as lymphokines.

One of the ways echinacea is thought to enhance lymphocyte function is by increasing the lymphocyte's ability to multiply when faced with a challenge. Lymphocytes are valuable resources. The body does not want to mobilize them unless they are really needed, but when they are needed it is important that they multiply rapidly to mount an effective defense. Echinacea is believed to push the lymphocytes into active duty as well as increase their ability to multiply. Next, echinacea may enhance their ability to form antibodies, increase production of the body's own antiviral compound, interferon, and promote secretion of lymphokines.

Echinacea actives lymphocytes

With increased B cell function, more viruses and other infecting organisms are tagged with antibodies so that the macrophage can identify them for complete destruction. In our analogy of the macrophages as "MPs" and the lymphocytes as judge (and jury), once the criminal has been charged, it is once again the job of the MPs to take him away. The difference here, however, is that the officer in this case is also responsible for the lethal injection and cremation!

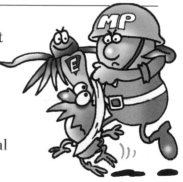

Echinamide helps the immune system "arrest" viruses and infections

Echinacea and the Killer Cells

The effect of echinacea on natural killer (NK) cells is particularly interesting.[13,14] As mentioned, these cells are extremely important in fighting against cancer and viral infections. Typically NK cell activity is reduced in individuals suffering from either chronic viral illness (such as chronic hepatitis or chronic fatigue syndrome) or cancer. Also, a decline in NK cell number or activity is also a common feature of aging. A recent study was designed to assess the numbers and production of NK cells in aging, normal mice, after administration of echinacea for 14 days, compared with the injection of thyroxin (thyroid hormone), a known stimulant of NK cell function.[13]

Results revealed that echinacea, but not thyroxin, had the capacity to increase NK cell numbers in aging mice. This suggests that echinacea increased new NK cell production in the bone marrow, leading to an increase in the absolute numbers of NK cells in the spleen, their primary destination. Echinacea's ability to increase NK cell numbers was paralleled by an increase

45

in their anti-tumor capacity. These results indicate that echinacea may also help boost NK cells in aging humans. Other studies have also shown enhanced NK cell activity and function with echinacea use.[14]

And for Our Next Trick...

Does echinacea have other effects on immunity? Yes, several. One of the most interesting and perhaps one of the first discovered effects of echinacea is its effect on the "complement system". This system is one of the body's first lines of defense and it acts like a sophisticated team of "reconnaissance" troops sent to patrol the battle zone looking for potential enemies.

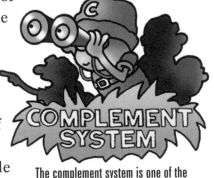

The complement system is one of the body's first lines of defense

The process of phagocytosis is an effective attack, but it takes time. So, the body also needs a faster acting attack force. It has one. This is the complement system—a system of about 20 different proteins secreted by the liver that can be activated to destroy infecting organisms and particulate matter. For example, one of the ways complement can destroy bacteria is by attaching itself to the invader in a way that sends a very powerful chemical signal out to monocytes (the blood macrophages) and neutrophils (those other white blood cell that engulf and destroy bacteria). This has an effect on the monocytes and neutrophils similar to waving a red flag at a bull. Other ways complement can destroy organisms is by poking holes in the organism's outer membrane, allowing water to rush in and important cellular components to rush out, causing the organisms to clump together (agglutinate).

Complement circulates in the blood looking for foreign material. In humans, cell surfaces contain special molecules that tell complement not to attack. Most organisms do not have these special molecules and the complement system considers them foreign invaders.

Echinacea and the Complement System

Echinacea affects the complement system both directly and indirectly. Echinacea enhances macrophage function and this automatically increases the production of complement because when macrophages are activated they send a signal to the liver to make more complement. Echinacea also directly increases the level of important complement system proteins in the blood.[10,15] So it is a double-effect that enhances the likelihood of a successful quick response to an infecting organism. The effect on the

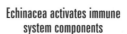

Echinacea activates immune system components

complement system is probably one of the key reasons why echinacea, and especially Echinamide, is most effective against the common cold if treatment is started at the first hint of a cold.

Echinacea Versus Viruses

Is echinacea antiviral? Yes. Various echinacea components have been shown to possess antiviral activity against the influenza, herpes and viruses that can cause the common cold.[16] However, although echinacea components may exhibit direct antiviral effects, the primary antiviral effects of echinacea may be due to the herb's ability to increase levels of the body's own antiviral forces.

Echinacea seems to increase production of a compound known as interferon and it helps inhibit an enzyme called hyaluronidase. This enzyme is secreted by the virus and "inhibited" by cichoric acid.[17] Hyaluronidase was originally known as the "spreading factor" because many organisms secrete it to breakdown connective tissue or intracellular "cement" that hold our cells together. Hyaluronic acid is an important structural component in our cells. The hyaluronidase enzyme dissolves the hyaluronic acid. Imagine your house having its doors and windows dissolved. That is similar to the result produced by the enzyme on connective tissue as it dramatically increases the permeability and allows the organism to anchor itself in the body.

Interestingly, echinacea was historically used for the treatment of snake bites. Although there have been no clinical studies to investigate this application, it has been reputed to be quite helpful. What is interesting about this folk use is the fact that most snake venoms permeate the system

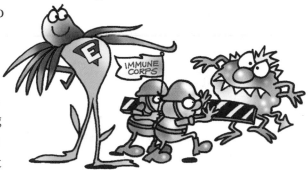

It seems that echinacea increases the effectiveness of the body's anti-viral squad

as a result of hyaluronidase in the venom breaking down the connective tissue substance. The bottom line here, in regards to echinacea's antiviral effects, is that by inhibiting hyaluronidase and generally enhancing immunity, echinacea is probably more effective against viruses than if it relied on its own antiviral activity.

Echinacea Against the Yeast Beast

Echinacea polysaccharides have also been shown to inhibit Candida albicans infection in rats infected intravenously with a lethal dose of Candida albicans.[18] The effect of echinacea against C. albicans noted in animal studies has been confirmed in several clinical studies. One study demonstrated that echinacea greatly enhances the effectiveness of a topical anti-yeast agent (ketoconazol nitrate) decreasing recurrence from 60.5% to 16.7%. The researchers used standardized skin tests to show that this enhancement was due to echinacea's boosting of cell-mediated immunity.[19]

Echinamide: Beyond Immunity

Besides being a fantastic ally of the immune system, echinacea has been particularly valued for its wound healing properties. This is due to its ability to promote tissue regeneration and reduce inflammation.[20,21] In addition to its effects on hyaluronidase (this enzyme will also be released by the body's own cells during an inflammatory process), echinacea also stimulates the growth of cells known as fibroblasts. These cells are responsible for the manufacture of the intracellular cement substance discussed earlier. In particular, echinacea has been shown to increase the manufacture of structural molecules critical in wound healing.[22]

Another interesting effect of echinacea involves enhancing the functioning of the adrenal glands, indicating that echinacea may be useful in helping us deal with stressful events more effectively.[23] Clinical studies indicate that echinacea can help prevent stress-induced suppression of immune function. While it is generally thought that the primary effect is due to echinacea's enhancement of immune function, this action on the adrenal glands may also play an important role.

Show Me the Studies

More than 30 clinical studies have been done with echinacea preparations. Most of these studies involved the prevention and treatment of the common cold and used fresh-pressed juice from the above-ground (aerial) portion of the *E. purpurea* plant, along with 22 percent ethanol (for preservation). Unfortunately, this form of echinacea is probably not the most beneficial because it has lower concentrations of key immune enhancing. Furthermore, as previously stated, there was no standardization in the levels of active compounds for any of the echinacea products used in these studies. This fact makes analysis very difficult and very nearly invalidates the results.

Nonetheless, numerous clinical studies have confirmed echinacea's immune enhancing actions. Various echinacea extracts or products have shown results in general infectious conditions, influenza, colds, upper respiratory tract infections, urogenital infections, and other infectious conditions.

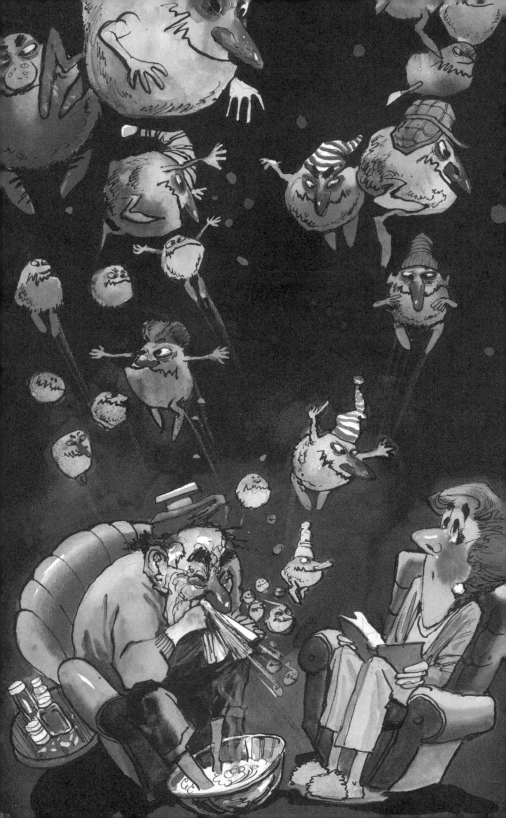

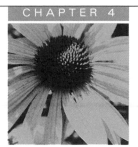

CHAPTER 4

IS THIS THE END OF THE COMMON COLD?

O ver the years, research results have been difficult to interpret because of the lack of quality control in preparations used. Simply stated, although most studies showed positive results, overall the results have been mixed. Some studies showed positive results in both preventing and treating the common cold, others showed little or no effect.[24-27] The reason for the mixed results is most likely due to the lack of consistency in the product being used. If the product, by chance, had sufficient levels of active compounds it would be effective. If not, then it would likely be no more effective than a placebo.

Weak Science = Questionable Results

Let me give you an example of the problems when looking at these studies in a superficial manner. In fact, it seems that a continuing trend in the evaluation of natural medicines is to design studies where the outcome will surely be negative and then using the results to launch a media campaign that makes gross generalizations. In the last few years the media have reported several studies as showing "echinacea is not effective", just as they have reported the "ineffectiveness" of other well known and trusted natural medicines. Of course, the real details of the studies were not given. Let's examine one such questionable study.[28]

A double blind, placebo-controlled study was conducted with 302 volunteers from 4 military institutions and 1 industrial plant in Germany. The subjects were given either a placebo, or alcohol-based tinctures from either *E. purpurea* or *E. angustifolia* for twelve weeks. The main outcome measured was time until the first upper respiratory tract infection. Secondary outcome measures were the number of participants with at least one infection, global assessment, and adverse effects. The time until occurrence of the first upper respiratory tract infection was 66 days in the *E. angustifolia* group, 69 days in the *E. purpurea* group, and 65 days in the placebo group. In the placebo group, 36.7 percent had an infection while in the *E. angustifolia* it was 32 percent and in the *E. purpurea* it was 29.3 percent. These results seem to indicate that there was no real significant benefit with either form of echinacea although there was an approximately 20 percent reduced risk of infection in the echinacea groups. In addition, 70 percent of the *E. purpurea* and 78 percent of the *E. angustifolia* group felt they had benefited from treatment compared to 56 percent in the placebo group. The *E. angustifolia* group had a slightly higher percentage of subjects experiencing side effects (18 percent) compared to the *E. purpurea* (10 percent) and placebo (11 percent) groups.

On the surface, these results do not seem to support the effectiveness of echinacea preparations in the prevention of upper respiratory infections. However, it is important to examine the form and dosage of the echinacea products used in this study. Both echinacea preparations used were very weak ethanol based tinctures. The herb to solvent ratio was 1:11 meaning that for every gram of herbal material there was 11 ml of the water and alcoholic (30% ethanol) solution. The dosage administered was 50 drops twice daily for a total of approximately 2 ml. Using the herb-to-solvent ratio, that represent about 200 mg of echinacea—hardly a therapeutic dose.

Furthermore, the starting material of both forms of echinacea was dried root, and neither preparation was analyzed for active compounds. If they had been analyzed, it is unlikely that either would have contained sufficient levels of actives to produce an effect.

So, take a low dosage of a poorly prepared, weak solution and you won't stop respiratory infections. What did the researchers expect? Very little and that is exactly what was demonstrated.

Quality Control for Immune Effectiveness

The problem of quality control with echinacea is possibly greater than any other plant for several reasons. Prior to Natural Factors' development of Echinamide there was not a product available that was standardized to contain all of the active compounds necessary for the complete, synergistic action of echinacea.

Some manufacturers may not even be using authentic sources of echinacea. For example, it has been estimated that, due to supplier errors in collection, more than 50 percent and possibly much as 90 percent of the echinacea sold in the US from 1908 through 1991 was actually another plant! Parthenium integrifolium. Like echinacea, Parthenium integrifolium has been referred to by the common name "Missouri snakeroot". In spite of possible confusion over the common names, these plants look quite different. Even though the root of *Parthenium integrifolium* when it is cut and sifted looks a lot like echinacea roots, it possesses a much different aroma. Of course, if manufacturers would bother to do even very simple chemical analyses, there would be no mistaking the two plants. Unfortunately, many manufacturers do not do any of their own quality control analysis.

Echinacea products are available in many different forms: ground or powdered crude herb, freeze-dried, alcohol-based tinctures and liquid extracts, aqueous tinctures and liquid extracts, and dry powdered alcoholic or aqueous extracts.

Are these forms effective? Remember what was stated above, *"What determines the effectiveness of any herbal product is its ability to deliver an effective dosage of active compounds."* If a manufacturer does not analyze for all of the key active compounds in their product, the consumer has no assurance that the product will produce the desired result.

Echinamide: The World's Best Echinacea

Natural Factors' testing and manufacturing procedures go beyond established guidelines to ensure the highest quality and consistency of product. Natural Factors grows their own echinacea using certified organic methods, hand weeding and harvesting with no chemical pesticides or herbicides, and the company's own laboratories analyze the plant material fresh from the field. These sophisticated labs use equipment such as HPLC (high pressure liquid chromatography)—a way to measure plant components at every stage of growth — to help determine the best harvesting time and extraction methods. All this attention to testing allows Natural Factors to produce a consistent Echinamide extract standardized for the three key active compounds.

Even after the finished product is complete, Natural Factors is not done testing because they want to ensure that the product is stable on the shelves of local natural health food stores and active when the consumer uses it. It is this attention to detail and dedication to quality that sets Echinamide and Natural Factors above all others.

Echinacea has been shown to exert significant effects on immune function in over 300 scientific investigations. Several classes of compounds are responsible for these effects. In order for an echinacea product to produce reliable and consistent results, it must contain a reliable and consistent amount of all of the active compounds of echinacea. Mixed results from clinical studies with echinacea are most likely due to lack of quality control in the product being used.

Appropriate quality control steps are absolutely essential in guaranteeing an effective product. Ultimately what determines the effectiveness of any herbal product is its ability to deliver an effective dosage of active compounds. The best assurance for consumers is to use a product that guarantees an effective dosage by guaranteeing the level of active ingredients.

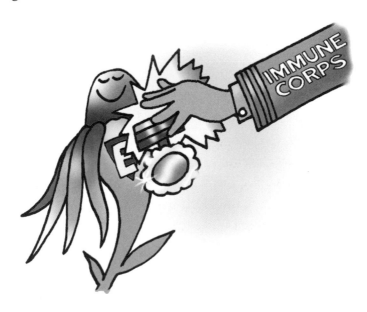

Echinamide is proven to enhance immunity

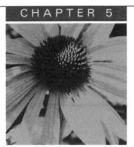

CHAPTER 5

Additional Natural Immune Support

The common cold is caused by a wide variety of viruses capable of infecting the upper respiratory tract – the nasal passages, sinuses, and throat – causing symptoms that are all too familiar; a general malaise, fever, headache and upper respiratory tract congestion. Initially there is a watery nasal discharge and sneezing followed by thicker secretions containing mucous, white blood cells, and dead organisms. The throat may be red, sore, and quite dry.

We are all constantly exposed to many of these viruses, yet the majority of us only experience the discomfort of a "cold" once or twice a year at the most. This suggests that a decrease in resistance or immune function is the major factor in "catching" a cold. In my opinion, maintaining a healthy immune system is the best way to protect yourself against an excessive number of colds. If you catch more than one or two colds per year, you may have a weakened immune system. In addition to Echinamide, there are other natural measures you can use to strengthen your immune system and help prevent colds and viral attacks, as well as speed recovery if you catch them, or they catch you.

What is the difference between a cold and the flu?

Usually a cold can be distinguished from other conditions with some similar symptoms (influenza and allergies for example) by some common sense. Influenza is much more severe in symptoms and usually occurs in epidemics, so contacting the local Public Health Department is all that is needed to rule this out. Allergies may be an underlying factor in decreasing resistance and allowing a virus to infect the upper airways, but usually allergies can be differentiated from the common cold by the fact that no fever occurs with allergies. There is also usually a history of seasonal allergic episodes with no evidence of infection.

What determines the health of the immune system?

The health of the immune system is greatly affected by a person's emotional state, level of stress, lifestyle, dietary habits and nutritional status. Nutrient deficiency is the most frequent cause of a depressed immune system. An overwhelming number of clinical and experimental studies indicate that any single nutrient deficiency can profoundly impair the immune system.

What dietary factors are important in immune support?

Consistent with overall good health, optimal immune function requires a healthy diet rich in whole, natural foods, such as fruits, vegetables, grains, beans, seeds, and nuts; low in fats and refined sugars, and containing adequate, but not excessive, amounts of protein. Dietary factors that depress immune function include nutrient deficiency, excess consumption of sugar, and consumption of allergenic foods.

What nutritional supplements can I take for immune system support?

A high-potency multiple-vitamin and mineral formula is the first step in supporting the immune system with nutritional supplementation as it will address any underlying nutritional deficiencies. Deficiencies of virtually any nutrient can result in significantly impaired immune function especially deficiencies of vitamins C, E, A, B6, B12, and folic acid. Minerals that are especially important are zinc, iron, and selenium. In addition to a multiple, some specific nutrients are particularly helpful in boosting immune function: vitamin C, vitamin E, and vitamin A.

Vitamin C (ascorbic acid) plays an important role in the immune system. Many different immune-enhancing effects have been demonstrated, including enhancing white blood cell response and function, increasing interferon (a special chemical factor that fights viral infection and cancer) levels, and improving the integrity of the linings of mucous membranes. Numerous clinical studies support the use of vitamin C in the treatment of infectious conditions, particularly the common cold. Vitamin C levels are quickly depleted during the stress of an infection. The recommended level for immune building is 500 to 1,000 mg one to three times daily. It is useful to take vitamin C with an equal amount of bioflavonoids since these compounds raise the concentration of vitamin C in some tissues and increase its beneficial effects.

Vitamin E exerts very good immune-enhancing activity. Even without signs of vitamin E deficiency, supplementation with vitamin E has been shown to exert a number of positive effects on immune functions. The benefits of vitamin E are especially helpful in enhancing immune function in the elderly. The recommended dosage is 400 to 800 IU of natural source vitamin E (d-alpha tocopherol).

Vitamin A was once known as the "anti-infective vitamin" and has recently regained recognition as a major determinant of immune status. Vitamin A affects the immune system in several ways. Primarily, it plays an essential role in maintaining the surfaces of the skin, respiratory tract, gastrointestinal tract, and other body tissues as well as their secretions. These surface systems constitute a primary barrier to microorganisms. In addition to this role, vitamin A has been shown to stimulate and/or enhance numerous immune processes, including induction of anti-tumor activity, enhancement of white blood cell function, and increased antibody response. Vitamin A has also demonstrated significant antiviral activity and has prevented the immune suppression induced by adrenal hormones, severe burns, and surgery. During an acute viral infection, a single oral dose of 50,000 IU for one or two days appears to be safe even for infants. In general, however, the daily dosage of vitamin A for immune support should be 5,000 to 10,000 IU. Beta carotene can be used instead and may offer some benefits greater than vitamin A.

Beta carotene has demonstrated a number of immune-enhancing effects in recent studies separate from its conversion to vitamin A. The recommended level of beta carotene for immune support is 25,000 to 50,000 IU (15 to 30 mg).

WARNING: Vitamin A supplementation must be absolutely avoided during pregnancy as it can lead to birth defects. Women who are at risk for becoming pregnant or are pregnant should keep their supplemental vitamin A levels below 5,000 IU or, better yet, use beta-carotene.

What herbs other than echinacea are useful or supporting the immune system?

Ecinacea is the most widely used Western herb for enhancement of the immune system while in Chinese medicine this title goes to Astragalus root. Clinical studies in China have shown it to be effective when used as a preventive measure against the common cold.30,31 It has also been shown to reduce the duration and severity of symptoms in acute treatment of the common cold, as well as raise white blood cell counts in chronic leukopenia (a condition characterized by low white blood cell levels). The dosage of the dried root is 1,000 to 2,000 mg three times daily. The dosage for astragalus extract (0.5% 4-hydroxy-3-methoxy isoflavone) is 100–150 mg three times daily.

Natural Factors has an excellent *Anti-Viral Formula*, developed by Dr. Mark Stengler and Dr. Jan

V. Slama, that contains Echinamide with extracts of astragalus, reishi mushroom, lomatium and licorice root. In addition to enhancing immune function, these additional herbs all have demonstrated antiviral activity. In Canada, the product is called Anti-Viral Formula while in the US it is called "Anti-V".

Does a person's mood or attitude affect immune function

Our mood and attitude have a tremendous bearing on the function of our immune system. The bottom line is that when we are happy and optimistic, our immune system functions much better. Conversely, when we are depressed, our immune system tends to be depressed. When a person is under more stress or is depressed, they will need to make a conscious effort to boost their immune system—that includes taking their supplements. It is not only major life stresses that can cause depressed immune function, but the more significant the stressor the greater the impact on the immune system. Negative emotions suppress immune function while positive emotions enhance immune function. In my clinical practice, whenever a patient is suffering from low immune function I will ask them who their favorite comedian is and then write a prescription for them to watch a movie or TV show that features that comedian.

What do I do once I catch a cold?

Once a cold develops there are several things that can speed up recovery. Do not expect immediate relief in most instances when using natural substances. In fact, since most natural therapies for colds involve assisting the body rather than the familiar drug action of suppressing the symptoms. So often the symptoms of the cold can temporarily worsen when using natural remedies. How can this be? Many of the symptoms of the cold are a result of our body's defense mechanisms. For example, the potent immune stimulating compound interferon released by our blood cells and other tissues during infections is responsible for many flu-like symptoms.

Another example is the beneficial effect of fever on the course of infection. While an elevated body temperature can be uncomfortable, suppression of fever is thought to counteract a major defense mechanism and prolong the infection. In general, fever should not be suppressed during an infection unless it is dangerously high (>104°F). For these and other reasons it is not uncommon for the individual treating themselves for the common cold with natural medicines to experience a greater degree of discomfort due to the immune enhancing effects of these compounds. Of course the illness is generally much shorter lived.

Here are some basic recommendations that I am sure that you have heard before, but you may not have really understood why they are important:

Rest

The immune system functions better under the parasympathetic arm of our autonomic nervous system, the system that controls unconscious body functions. The parasympathetic arm assumes control over bodily functions during periods of rest, relaxation, visualization, meditation and sleep. During the deepest levels of sleep, potent immune enhancing compounds are released and many immune functions are greatly increased. The value of sleep and rest during a cold cannot be overemphasized. In contrast, the other arm of the autonomic nervous system, the sympathetic arm, takes control when we are under stress and is largely responsible for the so-called fight or flight response. Hormones, like adrenaline, released by the flight or fight response actually impair immune function. After all, you would not be too concerned about the common cold if you were being chased by a tiger. So, rest is an important recommendation to boost immune function.

Consume Liquids

Drink lots of fluids. Increased fluid consumption offers several benefits. When the membranes that line the respiratory tract get dehydrated it provides a much more hospitable environment for the virus. Consuming plenty of liquids and/or using a vaporizer maintain a moist respiratory tract that repels viral infection. Drinking plenty of liquids will also improve the function of white blood cells by decreasing the concentration of solutes in the blood.

It should be noted that the type of liquids consumed is very important. Studies have shown that consuming concentrated sources of sugars like glucose, fructose, sucrose, honey or orange juice greatly reduces the ability of the white blood cells to kill bacteria. Before being consumed, fruit juices should be greatly diluted. Drinking concentrated orange juice during a cold probably does more harm than good.

Avoid Sugar

As mentioned above, sugar consumption, even if derived from "natural" sources like fruit juices and honey, can impair immune functions. This impairment appears to be due to the fact that glucose (blood sugar) and vitamin C compete for transport sites into the white blood cells. Decreased vitamin C levels due to excessive sugar consumption may result in a significant reduction in white blood cell function.

Take Vitamin C

Many claims have been made about the role of vitamin C (ascorbic acid) in the prevention and

In 1975 Thomas Chalmers analyzed the possible effect of vitamin C on the common cold by calculating the average difference in the duration of cold episodes in vitamin C and control groups in seven placebo-controlled studies. He found that episodes were 0.11 days shorter in the vitamin C groups and concluded that there was no valid evidence to indicate that vitamin C is beneficial in the treatment of the common cold. Chalmers' review has been extensively cited in scientific articles and monographs. However, other reviewers have concluded that vitamin C significantly alleviates the symptoms of the common cold. A careful analysis of Chalmers' review reveals serious shortcomings. For example, Chalmers did not consider the amount of vitamin C used in the studies and included in his meta-analysis was a study in which only 25-50 mg/day of vitamin C was administered to the test subjects! For some studies Chalmers used values inconsistent with the original published results. Using data from the same studies, the authors of the new study calculated that vitamin C at a dosage of 1-6 g/day decreased the duration of the cold episodes by nearly a full day — or roughly by 21%. The argument in the medical literature that vitamin C has no effect on the common cold seems to be based in large part on a faulty review written two decades ago.

treatment of the common cold. It has been over 20 years since Linus Pauling wrote the book *Vitamin C and the Common Cold*. Pauling based his opinion on several studies that showed vitamin C was very effective in reducing the severity of symptoms as well as the duration of the common cold. Since 1970, there have been over 20 double-blind studies designed to test Pauling's assertion. However, despite the fact that every study demonstrated that the group receiving the vitamin C had either a decrease in duration or symptom severity, for some reason the clinical effect is still debated in the medical community. A 1995 article that appeared in the *Journal of the American College of Nutrition* has shed some light on the controversy.[32]

Use Zinc Lozenges

One of the most popular natural approaches to the common cold is the use of zinc lozenges. There is good scientific data to support this practice as several studies have now shown that zinc lozenges provide relief of a sore throat due to the common cold. Zinc is a critical nutrient for optimum immune system function and, like vitamin C, zinc also possesses direct antiviral activity. There have been several double-blind, placebo controlled studies showing the benefits of zinc lozenges in reducing the severity and duration of cold symptoms. In one of the most recent studies, one hundred patients experiencing the early signs of the common cold were provided a lozenge which contained either 13.3 mg of zinc (from zinc gluconate) or placebo. They took the lozenges as long as they had symptoms.[33]

The subjects kept track of symptoms such as cough, headache, hoarseness, muscle ache, nasal drainage, nasal congestion, scratchy throat, sore throat, sneezing, and fever (assessed by oral temperature). The time to complete resolution of symptoms was significantly shorter in the zinc group than in the placebo group. Complete recovery was achieved in 4.4 days with zinc compared with 7.6 days for the placebo. The zinc group also had significantly fewer days with coughing (2.0 days compared with 4.5 days), headache (2.0 days vs 3.0 days), hoarseness (2.0 days vs 3.0 days), nasal congestion (4.0 days vs 6.0 days), nasal drainage (4.0 days vs 7.0 days), and sore throat (1.0 day vs 3.0 days).

Despite these promising results, it appears that not all zinc lozenges are effective. A few early studies did not show much benefit from zinc lozenges. This inconsistency was probably due to an ineffective lozenge formulation. It appears that in order for a zinc lozenge to be effective it must be free from sorbitol, mannitol and citric acid. The best lozenges are those that use glycine as the sweetener. Use lozenges supplying 15 to 25 mg of elemental zinc. Dissolve in the mouth every two waking hours after an initial double dose. Continue for up to 7 days.

Take Echinamide

Echinamide provides the best way to gain all of the benefits that echinacea has to offer in the fight against the common cold. Echinamide is available in several different forms. Here are my recommendations on which form is best for you along with dosage recommendations:

For example, in addition to the Echinamide *Anti-Viral Formula* described on page 64 , there are Echinamide products designed specifically for infants and children (e.g., Big Friends Echinamide); coughs and colds (Echinamide Cough & Cold Syrups); and extra strength Echinamide products available in capsules, alcohol-based tinctures and fluid extracts, alcohol-free liquids and syrups, and as throat sprays.

For general use to boost immune function, follow the dosage recommendations on the label. However, when dealing with a cold or flu, you will need to start with a "loading dosage." Basically, double the dosage amount stated on the bottle and take it every two to three waking hours during the first 48 hours of use. (Note: This recommendation does not apply to the Echinamide Cold Formulas that contain ephedra.) For example, the dosage recommendation on the label for Echinamide Extra Strength Tincture is 12 drops two times per day in a glass of water. During the first 48 hours of use, the loading dosage would then be 24 drops in water every two to three hours.

Although the focus of this chapter was on the use of natural methods to assist the body in recovering from the common cold, prevention is by far the best medicine. The old adage "an ounce of prevention is worth a pound of cure" is true for the common cold as well as the majority of other conditions afflicting human health. Once a cold catches you, here are my key recommendations:

- Rest (bed rest is best)

- Drink large amounts of fluids (preferably diluted vegetable juices, soups, and herb teas)

- Limit simple sugar consumption (including fruit sugars) to less than 50 grams a day

- Vitamin C: 500 to 1,000 mg every two hours (decrease if it produces excessive gas or diarrhea) along with 1,000 mg of mixed bioflavonoids per day

- Zinc lozenges: The best lozenges are those which utilize glycine as the sweetener. Use lozenges supplying 15 to 25 mg of elemental zinc. Dissolve in the mouth every two waking hours after an initial double dose. Continue for up to 7 days. Prolonged supplementation (more than one week) at this dose is not recommended as it may lead to suppression of the immune system.

- Echinamide: Follow recommendations given on these pages.

ECHINAMIDE

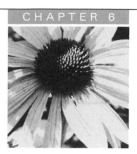

CHAPTER 6

Common Questions and Answers on echinacea and Echinamide

Should echinacea be taken on a daily basis?

The question whether echinacea should be used on a long-term or continual basis has not been adequately answered. The usual recommendation with long-term use is 8 weeks on followed by one week off. Research suggests that the people most likely to benefit from using echinacea for prevention are those with weaker immune systems who are more prone to infection. Therefore I do not recommend echinacea as a daily preventative measure for people with healthy immune function unless they are facing increased exposure to viruses or stress.

Is echinacea safe?

Echinamide is extremely safe. When echinacea is used at the recommended doses even for indefinite periods, there is no danger of toxicity as no studies have reported acute or chronic toxicity.[34] Echinacea use is usually without side effects, however, allergic reactions have been reported in people who are allergic to other members of plants in the daisy family (daisy, ragweed, marigolds, etc.).

Are there any people who should not use echinacea?

Many experts recommend that echinacea should not be used by people with acquired immunodeficiency syndrome (AIDS) or human-immunodeficiency virus (HIV) infection. Theoretically, echinacea use may lead to stimulation of viral replication of the virus as well. Although somewhat controversial, until more research is done, I think it wise to avoid echinacea use if you are infected with HIV.

Since echinacea can enhance immune function, it must not be used in people who have had organ transplants or who are taking drugs to purposely suppress the immune system like cyclophosphamide. This recommendation is based on the theoretical premise that echinacea may interfere with these drugs that are purposely used to suppress the immune system from rejecting the transplanted organ.

Can pregnant women use echinacea?

Echinacea appears to be safe even for pregnant or lactating women based upon both animal studies and evaluation studies in women using echinacea during pregnancy.[35]

What about children?

The general consensus among experts is that echinacea appears to be very safe even in very young children. For children under the age of six years, it is usually given at one-half the adult dosage.

Can people with autoimmune diseases take echinacea?

My recommendation is that people with autoimmune diseases such as rheumatoid arthritis, lupus, and multiple sclerosis avoid long-term use of echinacea. Taking echinacea for short periods of time is not likely to be a problem. The concern with echinacea in these conditions is that since they are characterized by an autoimmune reaction (a process in which antibodies formed by the immune system attack the body's own tissue), enhancing immune function may be harmful. My own opinion is that this may not be an issue as echinacea is more of an immune system modulator (normalizer) than stimulator. In fact, echinacea may ultimately be shown to be helpful for autoimmune diseases as uncontrolled studies have actually found it to be useful in rheumatoid arthritis.

Can echinacea be used in patients with cancer?

At this time the answer appears to be "yes" although more research is definitely needed. In animal studies, echinacea extracts have been shown to inhibit the growth of various cancers in experimental animal studies. In preliminary human studies, a stimulatory effects on white blood cell counts or function in patients receiving radiation or chemotherapy for cancer has been noted.[36,37]

Is echinacea helpful in fighting herpes infections?

Herpes simplex is a virus responsible for cold sores and genital herpes. There are two types of Herpes simplex viruses: type 1 (HSV-1) is most often responsible for cold sores (also referred to as fever blisters) while type 2 (HSV-2) is responsible for nearly 90 percent of cases of genital herpes. Slight differences between the viruses results in a preference for the location of infection. The sores known as lesions, develop as small red bumps and then turn into blisters or painful open sores. Over a period of days, the sores become crusted and then heal without scarring. Other symptoms can include fever, headache, muscle aches, painful or difficult urination, vaginal discharge, and swollen glands in the groin area. What preliminary studies indicate is that echinacea may contribute significantly to the faster healing of acute lesions, reduction of relapses, and prevention of initial infections.

Some companies claim echinacea angustifolia is better than E. purpurea. Is this claim true?

Not likely. *E. purpurea*, especially that used for Echinamide products, contains higher levels of three key ingredients: cichoric acid, alkylamides, and polysaccharides with immune enhancing properties.[2,38] Based upon currently available information, it appears that the best choice of echinacea is the above ground portion of *E. purpurea*.

Many companies claim their products are standardized for "total phenolic compounds" or echinacoside. Is this valid?

No. In fact, although these sort of echinacea extracts were found to have some antioxidant properties, recent studies have found them to have no effect on enhancing immune function in experimental animal studies.[1] Standardizing an echinacea preparation for these compounds alone does not mean it is an active product. It just highlights the importance of standardizing preparations for the three classes of active compounds responsible for the main immune enhancing effects– polysaccharides, cichoric acid, and alkylamides. Again, Echinamide is the only commercially available product that accomplishes this goal.

References

1   Rininger JA, Kickner S, Chigurupati P, et al.: Immunopharmacological activity of echinacea preparations following simulated digestion on murine macrophages and human peripheral blood mononuclear cells. *Leukoc Biol* 2000;68:503-10.

2   Bauer R: Standardization of echinacea purpurea expressed juice with reference to cichoric acid and alkamides. *J Herbs Spices Medicinal Plants* 1999;6:51-61.

3   Perry NB, van Klink JW, Burgess EJ, Parmenter GA: Alkamide levels in echinacea purpurea: effects of processing, drying and storage. *Planta Med* 2000;66:54-6.

4   Kim HO, Durance TD, Scaman CH, Kitts DD: Retention of alkamides in dried echinacea purpurea. *J Agric Food Chem* 2000;48:4182-92.

5   Luettig B, Steinmuller C, Gifford GE, et al.: Macrophage activation by the polysaccharide arabinogalactan isolated from plant cell cultures of echinacea purpurea. *J Nat Cancer Inst* 1989;81:669-75.

6   Vomel V: Influence of a non-specific immune stimulant on phagocytosis of erythrocytes and ink by the reticuloendothelial system of isolated perfused rat livers of different ages. *Arzneim Forsch* 1984;34.691-5.

7   Bauer R, Jurcic K, Puhlmann J, Wagner H: Immunological in vivo and in vitro examinations of echinacea extracts. *Arzneim Forsch* 1988;38:276-81.

8   Burger RA, Torres AR, Warren RP, et al.: Echinacea-induced cytokine production by human macrophages. *Int J Immunopharmacol* 1997;19:371-9.

9   Goel, V, Chang C, Slama JV, et al.: Dose related effects of echinacea on macrophage stimulation in lungs and in spleens of normal rats. *In press.*

10 Bauer R and Wagner H: Echinacea species as potential immuno-stimulatory drugs. *Econ Med Plant Res* 1991;5:253-321.

11 Wagner V, Proksch A, Riess-Maurer I, et al.: Immunostimulating polysaccharides (heteroglycans) of higher plants. *Arzneim Forsch* 1985;35:1069-75.

12 Stimpel M: Proksch A, Wagner H, Lohmann-Matthes ML: Macrophage activation and induction of macrophage cytotoxicity by purified polysaccharide fractions from the plant echinacea purpurea. *Infection Immunity* 1984;46;845-9.

13 Currier NL, Miller SC: Natural killer cells from aging mice treated with extracts from echinacea purpurea are quantitatively and functionally rejuvenated. *Exp Gerontol* 2000;35:627-39.

14 See DM, Broumand N, Sahl L, Tilles JG: In vitro effects of echinacea and ginseng on natural killer and antibody-dependent cell cytotoxicity in healthy subjects and chronic fatigue syndrome or acquired immunodeficiency syndrome patients. *Immunopharmacology* 1997;35:229-35.

15 Mose J: Effect of echinacin on phagocytosis and natural killer cells. *Med Welt* 1983;34:1463-7.

16 Wacker A, Hilbig W: Virus-inhibition by echinacea purpurea. *Planta Medica* 1978;33:89-102.

17 Facino RM, Carini M, Aldini G, et al.: Direct characterization of caffeoyl esters with antihyaluronidase activity in crude extracts from echinacea angustifolia roots by fast atom bombardment tandem mass spectrometry. *Farmaco* 1993;48:1447-61.

18 Roesler J, Steinmuller C, Kiderlen A, et al.: Application of purified polysaccharides from cell cultures of the plant echinacea purpurea to mice mediates protection against systemic infections with Listeria monocyto genes and Candida albicans. *Int J Immunopharmac* 1991;13:27-37.

19 Coeugniet EG, Kuhnast R: Recurrent candidiasis: adjuvant immunotherapy with different formulations of Echinacin. *Therapiewoche* 1986;36:3352-8.

20 Tubaro A, Tragni E, Del Negro P, et al.: Anti-inflammatory activity of a polysaccharide fraction of echinacea angustifolia root. *J Pharm Pharmacol* 1987;39:567-9.

21 Tragni E, Tubaro A, Melis S, Galli CL: Evidence from two classic irritation tests for an anti-inflammatory action of a natural extract, Echinacina B. *Food Chem Toxicol* 1985;23:317-9.

22 Tunnerhoff FK, Schwabe HK: Studies in human beings and animals on the influence of echinacea extracts on the formation of connective tissue following the implantation of fibrin.] *Arzneim Forsch* 1956;6:330-4.

23 Bonadeo I; Lavazza M: Echinacin B: Active polysaccharide of echinacea. *Riv Ital Essenze Profumi* 1971;53: 281–295.

24 Giles JT, Palat CT, Chien SH, et al.: Evaluation of echinacea for treatment of the common cold. *Pharmacotherapy.* 2000;20:690-7.